The Super Guide of

Diet for Carb L

Learn How to Lose Weight and Stay

Healthy with Tested Recipes from

Breakfast to Dinner.

Pamela Cooney

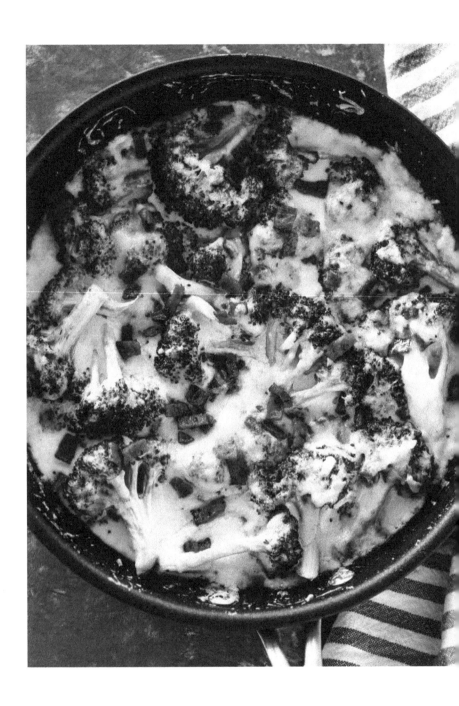

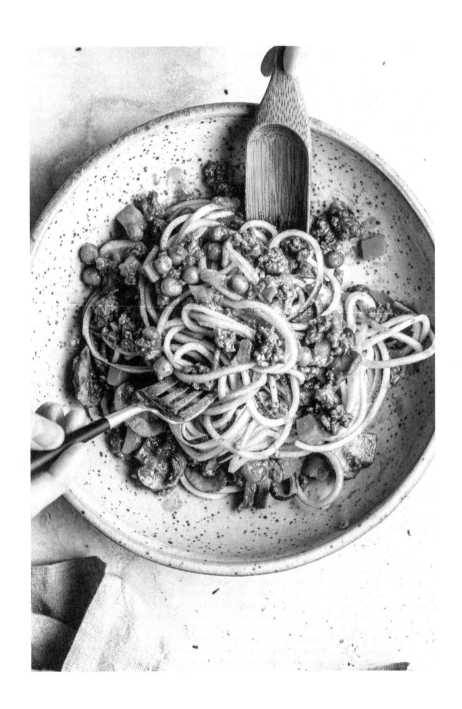

This declaration is deemed fair and valid by both the American Bar Association and the Committee of Publishers Association and is legally binding throughout the United States.

Furthermore, the transmission, duplication, or reproduction of any of the following work including specific information will be considered an illegal act irrespective of if it is done electronically or in print. This extends to creating a secondary or tertiary copy of the work or a recorded copy and is only allowed with the express written consent from the Publisher. All additional right reserved.

The information in the following pages is broadly considered a truthful and accurate account of facts and as such, any inattention, use, or misuse of the information in question by the reader will render any resulting actions solely under their purview. There are no scenarios in which the publisher or the original author of this work can be in any fashion deemed liable for any hardship or damages that may befall them after undertaking information described herein.

Additionally, the information in the following pages is intended only for informational purposes and should thus be thought of as universal. As befitting its nature, it is presented without assurance regarding its prolonged validity or interim quality. Trademarks that are mentioned are done without written consent and can in no way be considered an endorsement from the trademark holder.

Table of Contents

BREAKFAST

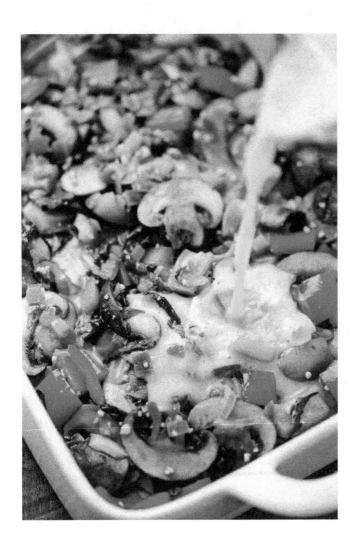

1.   Easy Beef Mushroom Stew

Preparation Time: 10 minutes

Cooking Time: 8 hours

Serves: 8

Ingredients:

- 2 lb. stewing beef, cubed

- 1packet dry onion soup mix

- 4oz. can mushrooms, sliced

- 14oz. can cream of mushroom soup

- 1/2cup water

- 1/4tsp. black pepper

- 1/2tsp. salt

Directions:

1. Spray a crock pot inside with cooking spray.

2. Add all ingredients into the crock pot and stir well.

3. Cover and cook on low for 8 hours.

4. Stir well and serve.

Nutrition: Calories 237 Fat 8.5 g Carbohydrates 2.7 g Protein: 31Sugar: 8

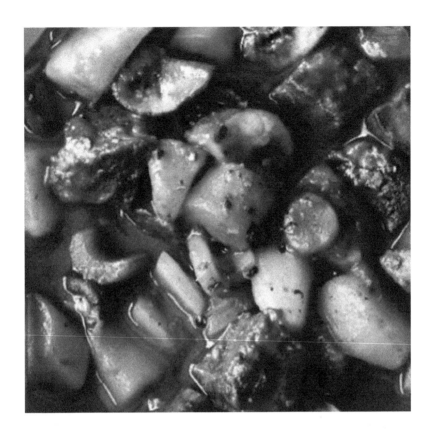

2. Lamb Stew

Preparation Time: 10 minutes

Cooking Time: 8 hours

Serves: 2

Ingredients:

- 1/2lb. lean lamb, boneless and cubed
- 2Tbsp. lemon juice
- 1/2onion, chopped
- 2garlic cloves, minced
- 2fresh thyme sprigs
- 1/4tsp. turmeric
- 1/4cup green olives, sliced
- 1/2tsp. black pepper
- 1/4tsp. salt

Directions:

1. Add all ingredients to a crock pot and stir well.
2. Cover and cook on low for 8 hours.
3. Stir well and serve.

Nutrition: Calories 297 Fat 20.3 g Carbohydrates 4.5 g Protein: 16Sugar: 3

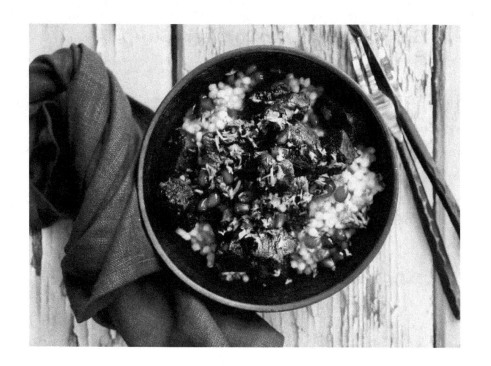

3. Vegetable Chicken Soup

Preparation Time: 10 minutes

Cooking Time: 6 hours

Serves: 6

Ingredients:

- 4cups chicken, boneless, skinless, cooked and diced
- 4tsp. garlic, minced
- 2/3cups onion, diced
- 11/2cups carrot, diced
- 6cups chicken stock
- 2Tbsp. lime juice
- 1/4cup jalapeño pepper, diced
- 1/2cup tomatoes, diced

- 1/ cup fresh cilantro, chopped

- 1tsp. chili powder

- 1Tbsp. cumin

- 13/4cups tomato juice

- 2tsp. sea salt

Directions:

1. Add all ingredients to a crock pot and

   stir well.

2. Cover and cook on low for 6 hours.

3. Stir well and serve.

Nutrition: Calories 192 Fat 3.8 g
Carbohydrates 3.8 g Protein: 13Sugar: 2

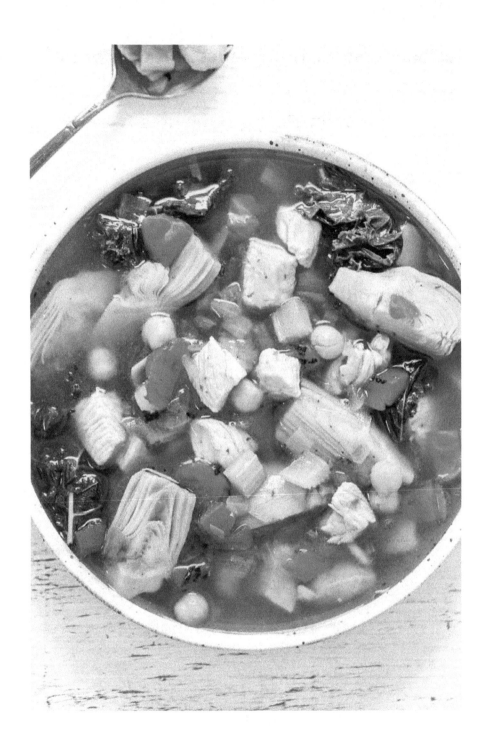

4.   Squash and Zucchini Casserole

Preparation Time: 10 minutes

Cooking Time: 6 hours

Serves: 6

Ingredients:

- 2cups yellow squash, quartered and sliced
- 2cups zucchini, quartered and sliced
- 1/4cup Parmesan cheese, grated
- 1/4cup butter, cut into pieces
- 1tsp. garlic powder
- 1tsp. Italian seasoning
- 1/4tsp. pepper
- 1/2tsp. sea salt

Directions:

1. Add sliced yellow squash and zucchini to a crock pot.

2. Sprinkle with garlic powder, Italian seasoning, pepper, and salt.

3. Top with grated cheese and butter.

4. Cover with the lid and cook on low for 6 hours.

5. Serve and enjoy.

Nutrition: Calories 107 Fat 9.5 g

Carbohydrates 2.5 g Protein: 14Sugar: 5

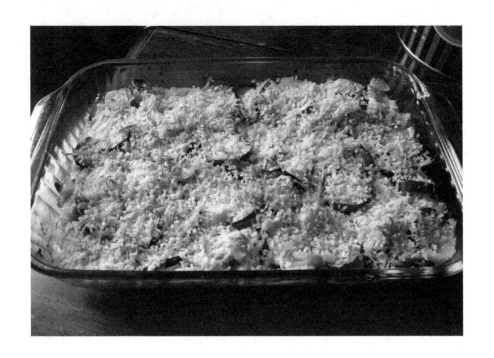

5.   Italian Zucchini

Preparation Time: 10 minutes

Cooking Time: 3 hours

Serves: 3

Ingredients:

- 2zucchini, cut in half lengthwise then cut into half moons
- 1/4cup Parmesan cheese, grated
- 1/2tsp. Italian seasoning
- 1Tbsp. olive oil
- 1Tbsp. butter
- 2garlic cloves, minced
- 1onion, sliced
- 2tomatoes, diced

- 1/2tsp. pepper

- 1/4tsp. salt

Directions:

1. Spray a crock pot inside with cooking spray.

2. Add all ingredients except Parmesan cheese to the crock pot and stir well.

3. Cover and cook on low for 3 hours.

4. Top with the Parmesan cheese and serve.

Nutrition: Calories 181 Fat 12.2 g Carbohydrates 1.2 g Protein: 17Sugar: 2

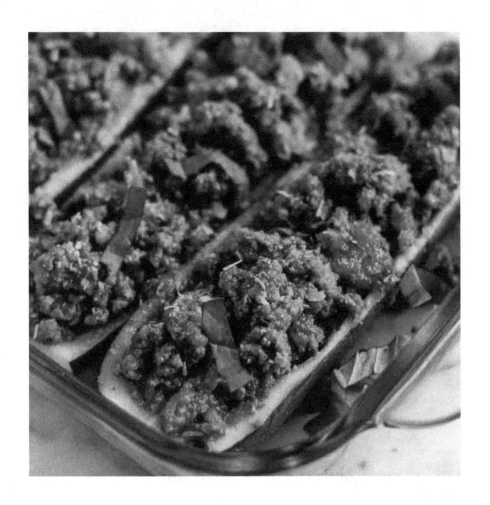

6.   Almond Green Beans

Preparation Time: 10 minutes

Cooking Time: 3 hours

Serves: 4

Ingredients:

- 1lb. green beans, rinsed and trimmed

- 1/2cup almonds, sliced and toasted

- 1cup vegetable stock

- 1/4cup butter, melted

- oz. onion, sliced

- 1Tbsp. olive oil

- 1/4tsp. pepper

- 1/2tsp. salt

Directions:

1. Heat the olive oil in a pan over medium heat.

2. Add onion to the pan and sauté until softened.

3. Transfer sautéed onion to a crock pot.

4. Add remaining ingredients except for almonds to the crock pot and stir well.

5. Cover and cook on low for 3 hours.

6. Top with toasted almonds and serve.

Nutrition: Calories 253 Fat 21.6 g Carbohydrates 4.5 g Protein: 21Sugar: 5

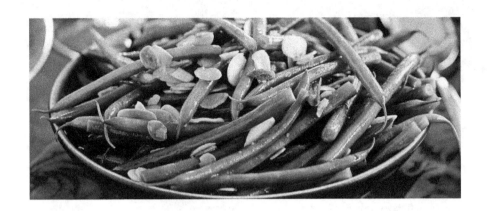

7.　Easy Ranch Mushrooms

Preparation Time: 10 minutes

Cooking Time: 3 Hours

Serves: 6

Ingredients:

- 2lb. mushrooms, rinsed, pat dry

- 2packets ranch dressing mix

- 3/4cup butter, melted

- 1/ cup fresh parsley, chopped

Directions:

1. Add all ingredients except parsley to a crock pot and stir well.

2. Cover and cook on low for 3 hours.

3. Garnish with parsley and serve.

Nutrition: Calories 237 Fat 23.5 g Carbohydrates 5 g Protein: 12Sugar: 8

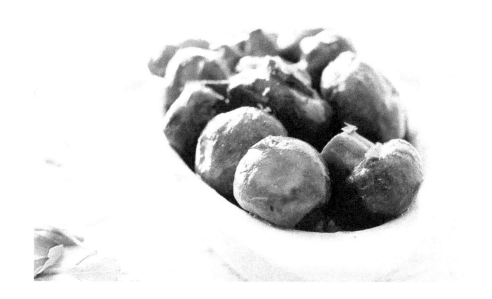

LUNCH

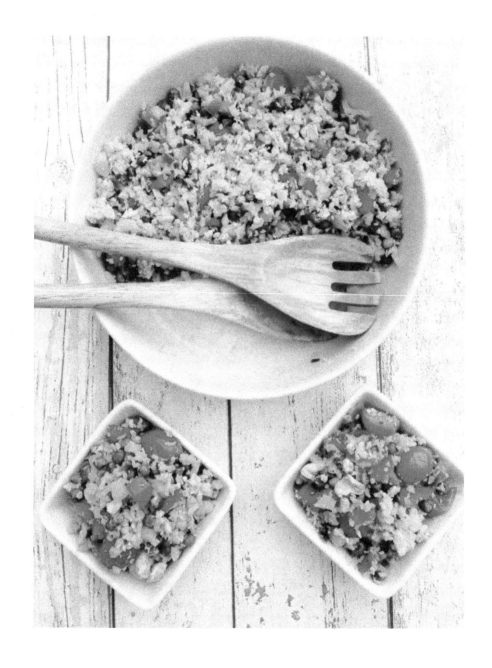

8. Cilantro Beef

Preparation time: 10 minutes

Cooking time: 4 hour

Servings: 2

Ingredients:

- 1-pound beef loin, roughly chopped
- 1/4cup apple cider vinegar
- 1tablespoon dried cilantro
- 1/2teaspoon dried basil
- 1 cup of water
- 1 teaspoon tomato paste

Direction

1. Mix meat with tomato paste, dried cilantro, and basil.
2. Then transfer it to the slow cooker.

3. Add apple cider vinegar and water.

4. Cook the cilantro beef for 4.5 hours on High. .

Nutrition: Calories 176 Fat 4 g Carbohydrates 1 g Sugar 4 g Protein 18

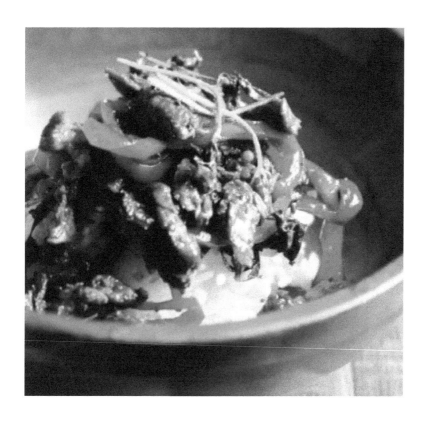

9. Potato Salad

Preparation time: 10 minutes

Cooking time: 3 hour

Servings: 2

Ingredients:

- 1cup potato, chopped

- 1 cup of water

- 1teaspoon salt

- 1oz. celery stalk, chopped

- 1oz. fresh parsley, chopped

- 1/4 onion, diced

- tablespoon mayonnaise

Directions:

1. Put the potatoes in the slow cooker.

2. Add water and salt.

3. Cook the potatoes on High for 3 hours.

4. Then drain water and transfer the potatoes in the salad bowl. 5 Add all remaining ingredients and carefully mix the salad.

Nutrition: Calories 165 Fat 13 g Carbohydrates 1.9 g Sugar 3 g Protein 28

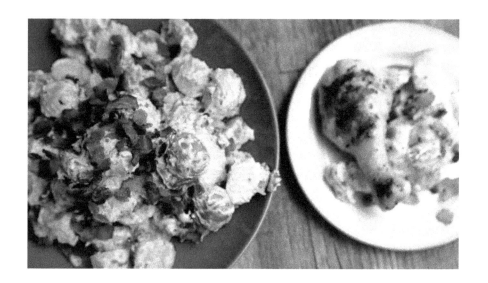

10.   Sautéed Greens

Preparation time: 15 minutes

Cooking time: 5 hour

Servings: 1

Ingredients:

- 1cup spinach, chopped

- water 2 cups

- collard greens, chopped

- 1/2 cup half and half

- 1 cup Swiss chard, chopped

Directions

1. Put spinach, collard greens, and Swiss chard in the slow cooker.

2. Add water and close the lid.

3. Cook the greens on High for 1 hour.

4. Then drain water and transfer the greens in the bowl.

5. Bring the half and half to boil and pour over greens.

6. Carefully mix the greens.

Nutrition: Calories 112 Fat 19 g Carbohydrates 1.9 g Sugar 3 g Protein 28

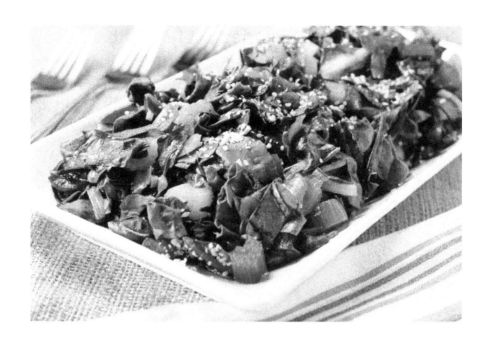

11. Mashed Turnips

Preparation time: 10 minutes

Cooking time: 7 hour

Servings: 2

Ingredients:

- 3-pounds turnip, chopped

- 2 cup water

- 1tablespoon vegan butter

- 1 tablespoon chives, chopped

- 1oz. Parmesan, grated

Directions

1. Add water and cook the vegetables on low for 7 hours. Then drain water and mash the turnips.

2. Add chives, butter, and Parmesan.

3. Carefully stir the mixture until butter and Parmesan are melted Then add chives. Mix the mashed turnips again.

Nutrition: Calories 198 Fat 19 g Carbohydrates 1.9 g Sugar 3 g Protein 12

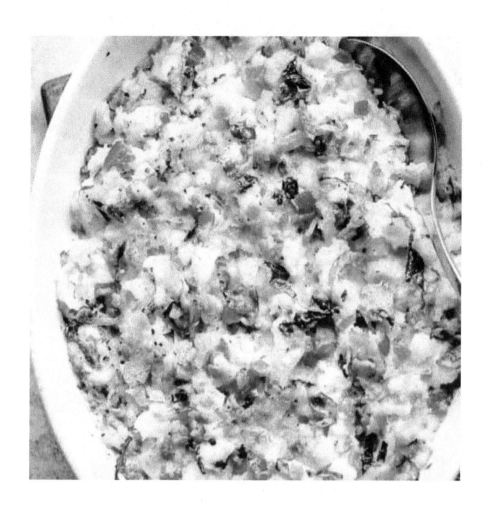

12.   Cilantro Meatballs

Preparation time: 20 minutes

Cooking time: 4 hour

Servings: 2

Ingredients:

- 1-pound minced beef
- 1 teaspoon minced garlic
- 1 egg, beaten
- 1teaspoon chili flakes
- 2teaspoons dried cilantro
- 1 tablespoon semolina
- 1/2 cup of water
- 1tablespoon sesame oil

Directions

1. In the bowl, mix minced beef, garlic, egg, chili flakes, cilantro, and semolina.

2. Then make the meatballs.

3. After this, heat the sesame oil in the skillet.

4. Cook the meatballs in the hot oil on high heat for 1 minute per side.

5. Transfer the roasted meatballs to the slow cooker, add water, and close the lid.

6. Cook the meatballs on High for 4 hours.

Nutrition: Calories 125 Fat 1 g Carbohydrates 3 g Sugar 3 g Protein 12

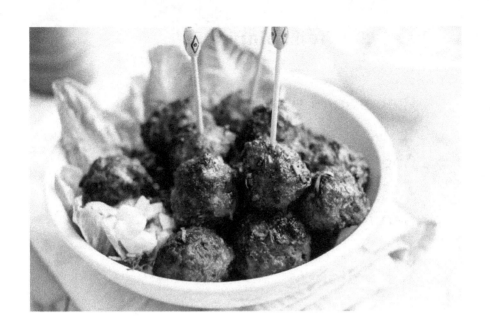

13. Stuffed Jalapenos

Preparation time: 10 minutes

Cooking time: 4 hour

Servings: 2

Ingredients:

- 1jalapenos, deseed
- 1oz. minced beef
- 1 teaspoon garlic powder
- 1/2 cup of water

Directions

1. Mix the minced beef with garlic powder.

2. Then fill the jalapenos with minced meat and arrange it in the slow

cooker. Add water and cook the jalapenos on High for 4.5 hours.

Nutrition: Calories 154 Fat 3 g Carbohydrates 5 g Sugar 2 g Protein 15

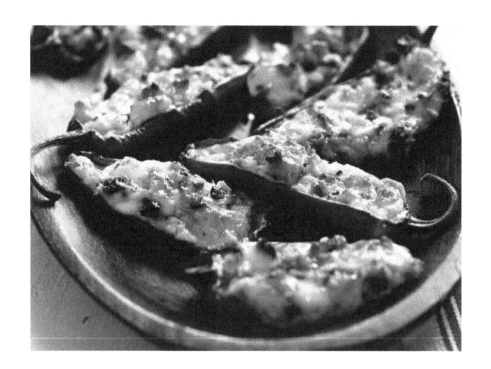

14.   BBQ Beef Short Ribs

Preparation time: 10 minutes

Cooking time: 5 hour

Servings: 2

Ingredients:

- 1-pound beef short ribs

- 1/3 cup BBQ sauce

- 1/4 cup of water

- 1 teaspoon chili powder

Directions

1. Rub the beef short ribs with chili powder and put in the slow cooker Mix water with BBQ sauce and pour

the liquid into the slow cooker. Cook

the meat on High for 5 hours.

Nutrition: Calories 187 Fat 2 g

Carbohydrates 1 g Sugar 4 g Protein 21

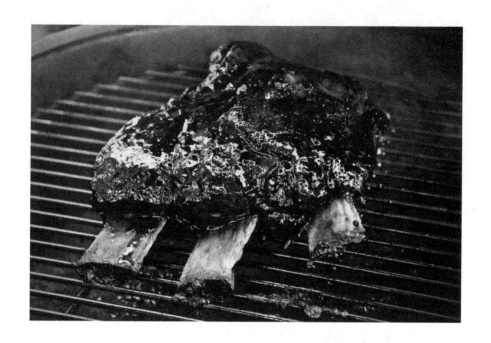

15.   Spiced Beef

Preparation time: 10 minutes

Cooking time: 9 hour

Servings: 2

Ingredients:

- 1-pound beef loin
- 1teaspoon allspice
- 1teaspoon olive oil
- 1 tablespoon minced onion
- 1 cup of water

Directions

1. Rub the beef loin with allspice, olive oil, and minced onion.

2. Put the meat in the slow cooker.

3. Add water and close the lid.

4. Cook the beef on Low for 9 hours.

5. When the meat is cooked, slice it into

servings.

Nutrition: Calories 187 Fat 2 g

Carbohydrates 1 g Sugar 4 g Protein 21

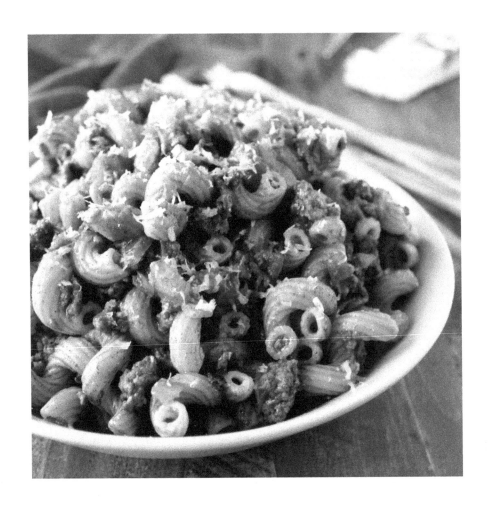

DINNER

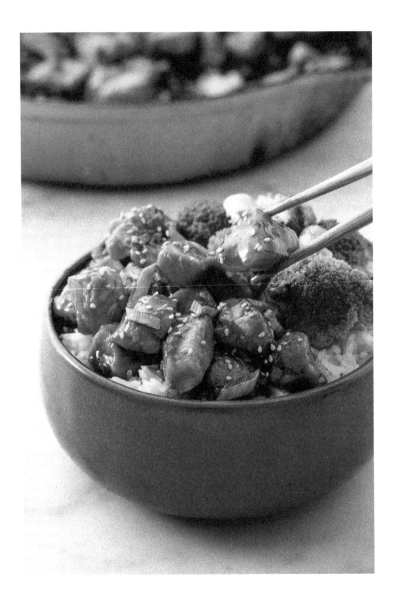

16. Sherry Chicken with Mashed Potatoes

Preparation Time: 5 minutes

Cooking time: 4 hrs.

Servings: 2

Ingredients

For the Sherry Chicken:

- 1/4 cup dry sherry
- 1cup raisins
- 4 medium-sized chicken breast
- 1 tart cooking apple, peeled and chopped
- 1 sweet onion, sliced

- 1 cup chicken broth

- Salt and pepper, to taste

- 2pounds Idaho potatoes, peeled and cooked

- 1/4 sour cream

- 1/3 cup whole milk

- 1/2tablespoons butter

- 1 teaspoon sea salt

- 1/4 teaspoon black pepper

- 1/4 teaspoon cayenne pepper

Directions

1. In a crock pot, place all of the ingredients for the sherry chicken; cover and cook on high until chicken breasts are tender or 3 to 4 hours.

2. Meanwhile, beat potatoes, adding sour cream, milk, and butter; beat until smooth and uniform.

3. Season with spices and serve on the side with sherry chicken.

Nutrition Calories: 154 Fat: 12 g Carbs: 3 g Protein: 15 g

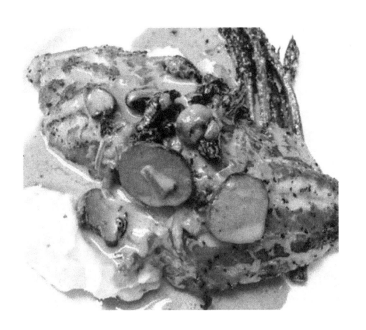

17. Kicked Up Chicken with Zucchini

Preparation Time: 5 minutes

Cooking time: 4 hrs.

Servings: 2

Ingredients

- 3 medium-sized chicken breasts, halved
- 1cup almond milk
- 1/4 cup water
- 1/4 cup lemon juice
- 2cloves garlic, minced
- 1 medium-sized onion, chopped
- Salt, to taste
- Red pepper, to taste

- 1 teaspoon ground ginger

- 1 teaspoon ground cumin

- 1 pound zucchini, sliced

- 1 tablespoon corn flour

- 1/2tablespoons water

- 1/3 cup fresh parsley, chopped

- 2cups rice, cooked

Directions

1. Place all ingredients, except zucchini, corn flour, water, parsley and rice, in your crock pot.

2. Cover and cook on low heat setting about 4 hours, adding zucchini during last 30 minutes of cooking time. Reserve chicken breasts.

3. Turn heat to high and continue cooking 10 minutes; stir in combined corn flour and water, stirring about 3 minutes.

4. Sprinkle with parsley; serve over rice.

Nutrition Calories: 265 Fat: 11 g Carbs:

3 g Protein: 15 g

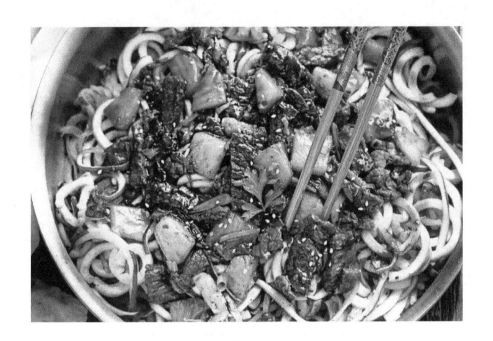

18. Festive Cornish Hens

Preparation Time: 5 minutes

Cooking time: 6 hrs.

Servings: 2

Ingredients

- 2 frozen Cornish hens, thawed

- 1/2 teaspoon sea salt

- 1/4 teaspoon ground black pepper

- 1/2 teaspoon cayenne pepper

- 2glove garlic, minced

- 1/3 cup chicken broth

- 1tablespoons corn flour

- 1/4 cup water

Directions

1. Sprinkle Cornish hens with salt, black pepper and cayenne pepper; add minced garlic and place in a crock pot. Pour in chicken broth.

2. Cover and cook on low 6 hours. Remove Cornish hens and reserve.

3. Stir in combined corn flour and water, stirring 2 to 3 minutes; serve.

Nutrition Calories: 234 Fat: 15 g Carbs:

2 g Protein: 12 g

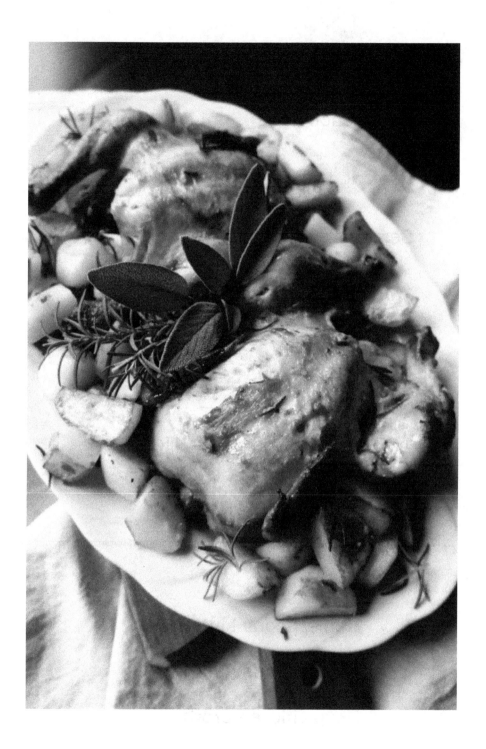

19. Salmon with Caper Sauce

Preparation Time: 5 minutes

Cooking time: 45 minutes.

Servings: 2

Ingredients

- 1/2 cup dry white wine

- 1/2 cup water

- 1yellow onion, thin sliced

- 1/2 teaspoon salt

- 1/4 teaspoon black pepper

- 4 salmon steaks

- 2tablespoons butter

- 2tablespoons flour

- 1 cup chicken broth

- 2 teaspoons lemon juice

- 3tablespoons capers

Directions

1. Combine wine, water, onion, salt and black pepper in a crock pot; cover and cook on high 20 minutes.

2. Add salmon steaks; cover and cook on high until salmon is tender or about 20 minutes.

3. To make the sauce, in a small skillet, melt butter over medium flame. Stir in flour and cook for 1 minute.

4. Pour in chicken broth and lemon juice; whisk for 1 to 2 minutes. Add capers; serve the sauce with salmon.

Nutrition Calories: 234 Fat: 15 g Carbs:

2 g Protein: 12 g

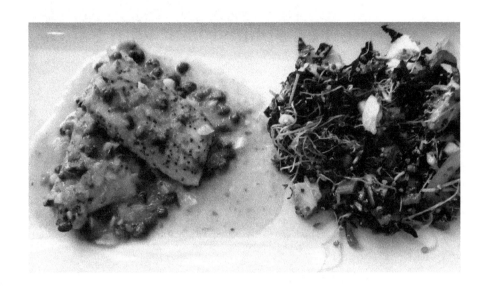

20. Herbed Salmon Loaf with Sauce

Preparation Time: 5 minutes

Cooking time: 5 hour.

Servings: 2

Ingredients

For the Salmon Meatloaf:

- 1cup fresh bread crumbs

- 1 can (7 1/2 ounce) salmon, drained

- 1/4 cup scallions, chopped

- 1/3 cup whole milk

- 1 egg

- 1 tablespoon fresh lemon juice

- 1 teaspoon dried rosemary

- 1 teaspoon ground coriander

- 1/2 teaspoon fenugreek

- 1 teaspoon mustard seed

- 1/2 teaspoon salt

- 1/4 teaspoon white pepper

- 1/2 cup cucumber, chopped

- 1/2 cup reduced-fat plain yogurt

- 1/2 teaspoon dill weed

- Salt, to taste

Directions

1. Line your crock pot with a foil.

2. Mix all ingredients for the salmon meatloaf until everything is well incorporated; form into loaf and place in the crock pot.

3. Cover with a suitable lid and cook on low heat setting 5 hours.

4. Combine all of the ingredients for the sauce; whisk to combine.

5. Serve your meatloaf with prepared sauce.

Nutrition Calories: 145 Fat: 11 g Carbs: 2 g Protein: 11 g

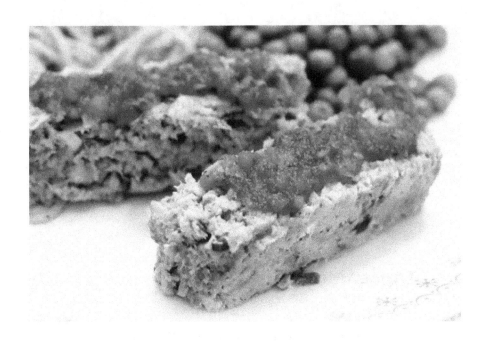

21.   Lazy Man Mac and Cheese

Preparation Time: 5 minutes

Cooking time: 5 hour.

Servings: 2

Ingredients

- Non-stick cooking spray-butter flavor

- 16 ounces macaroni of choice

- 1/2 cup butter, melted

- 1(12-ounce) can evaporated milk

- 1 cup milk

- 4 cups Colby jack cheese, grated

Directions

1. Lightly grease a crock pot with cooking spray.

2. First of all, cook your favorite macaroni according to package DIRECTIONS; rinse and drain; transfer to the crock pot.

3. Add the rest of ingredients and stir well. Cook on low heat setting 3 to 4 hours. Enjoy!

Nutrition Calories: 164 Fat: 11 g Carbs:

2 g Protein: 11 g

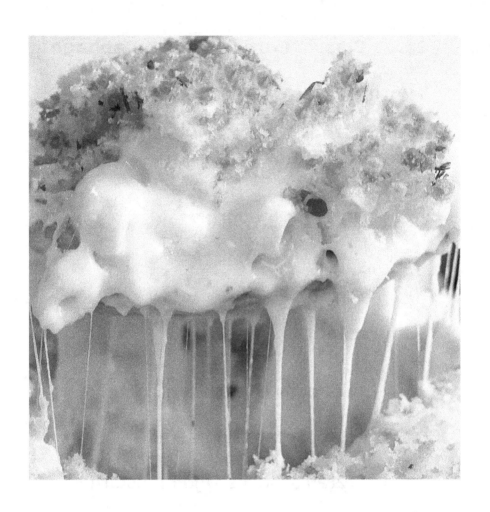

22. Classic Corned Beef & Cabbage with Horseradish Cream

Preparation Time: 10 minutes

Cooking time: 6 hour.

Servings: 2

Ingredients

- 11/2 cups sour cream
- 1cup prepared horseradish
- 1/2tablespoons Dijon mustard
- 11/2 teaspoons white wine vinegar
- 1 teaspoon kosher salt
- 1/2 teaspoon freshly ground black pepper

FOR THE BEEF

- 1 head cabbage, cut into wedges

- 1 onion, chopped

- 1/2 cup (1 stick) unsalted butter or Ghee (here), melted

- 11/2 cups water

- 1/2 teaspoon ground coriander

- 1/2 teaspoon ground mustard

- 1/2 teaspoon ground allspice

- 1/2 teaspoon ground marjoram

- 1/2 teaspoon ground thyme

- 1/2 teaspoon kosher salt

- 1/2 teaspoon freshly ground black pepper

- 1 (3-pound) corned beef brisket

Directions:

1. In a medium bowl, stir together all the ingredients. Cover and chill until ready to serve.

2. In the slow cooker, toss together the cabbage wedges, onion, and butter, and then spread them out in an even layer. Add the water.

3. In a small bowl, stir together the coriander, mustard, allspice, marjoram, thyme, salt, and pepper. Rub the spice mixture all over the corned beef. Place the beef on top of the vegetables in the slow cooker. Cover and cook for 8 hours on low.

4. Let the meat rest for 5 to 10 minutes before slicing. Serve with the vegetables and horseradish cream.

Nutrition Calories: 387 Fat: 11 g Carbs: 3 g Protein: 28 g

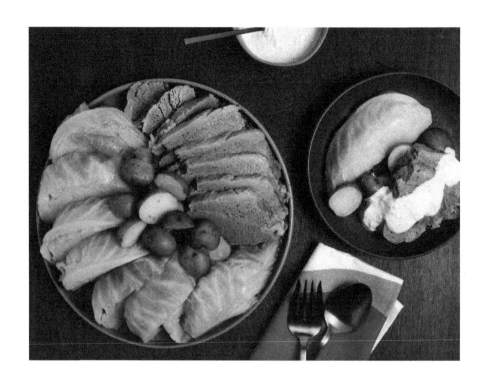

POULTRY RECIPES

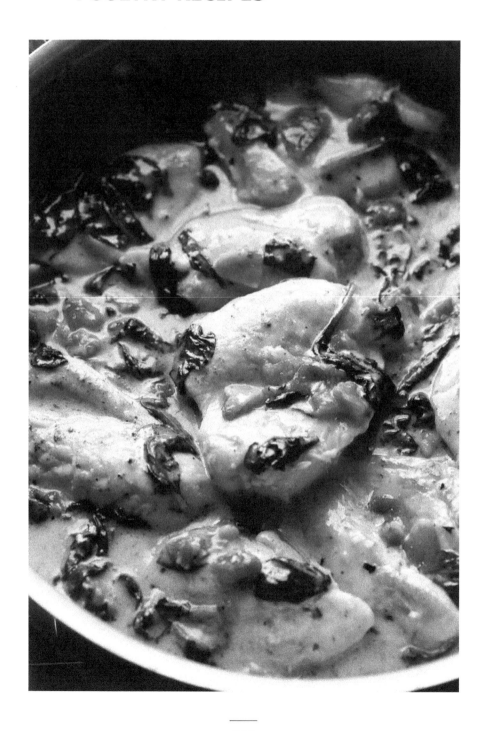

23. Greek Drumettes with Olives

Preparation time: 10 minutes

Cooking time: 20 minutes

Servings: 2

Ingredients:

- 1pound (454 g) chicken drumettes
- 1teaspoon Greek seasoning blend
- 1tablespoon olive oil
- ounces (170 g) tomato sauce
- Kalamata olives, pitted and sliced

Directions:

1. Place the chicken drumettes and Greek seasoning blend in a Ziploc

bag. Shake the bag, ensuring even coating.

2. Heat the olive oil in a saucepan over medium-high heat. Sear the chicken drumettes until golden brown, flipping them occasionally to ensure even cooking.

3. After that, stir in the tomato sauce and Kalamata olives. Continue to cook until the chicken is tender and everything is thoroughly heated or about 20 minutes. Bon appétit!

Nutrition: calories: 342 fat: 14.2g protein: 47.0g carbs: 3.5g net carbs: 2.4g fiber: 1.1g

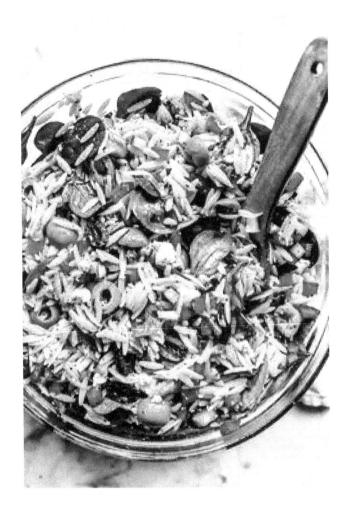

24. Tikka Masala

Preparation time: 10 minutes

Cooking time: 25 minutes

Servings: 2

Ingredients:

- 1½ pounds (680 g) chicken breasts, cut into bite-sized pieces
- 1onion, chopped
- 10 ounces (283 g) tomato purée
- 1teaspoon garam masala
- ½ cup heavy cream

Directions:

1. Heat a wok that is greased with a nonstick cooking spray over medium-

high heat. Now, sear the chicken breasts until golden brown on all sides.

2. Add the onions and sauté them for 2to 3 minutes more or until tender and fragrant. Stir in the tomato purée and garam masala. Cook for 10 minutes until the sauce turns into a dark red color.

3. Fold in the heavy cream and stir to combine. Cook for 10 to 13 minutes more or until heated through.

4. Serve with cauliflower rice if desired and enjoy!

Nutrition: calories: 293   fat: 17.1g

protein: 29.1g   carbs: 4.8g   net carbs:

3.6g fiber: 1.2g

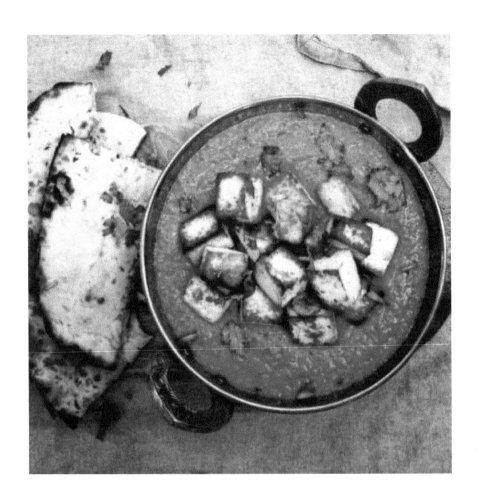

25. Simple White Wine Drumettes

Preparation time: 10 minutes

Cooking time: 35 minutes

Servings: 2

Ingredients:

- 1pound (454 g) chicken drumettes
- 1tablespoon olive oil
- 2tablespoons butter, melted
- 1garlic cloves, sliced
- Fresh juice of ½ lemon
- 2tablespoons white wine
- Salt and ground black pepper, to taste
- 1tablespoon fresh scallions, chopped

Directions:

1. Start by preheating your oven to 450ºF (235ºC). Place the chicken in a parchment-lined baking pan. Drizzle with olive oil and melted butter.

2. Add the garlic, lemon, wine, salt, and black pepper.

3. Bake in the preheated oven for about 35 minutes. Serve garnished with fresh scallions. Enjoy!

Nutrition: calories: 210 fat: 12.3g protein: 23.3g carbs: 0.5g net carbs: 0.4g fiber: 0.1g

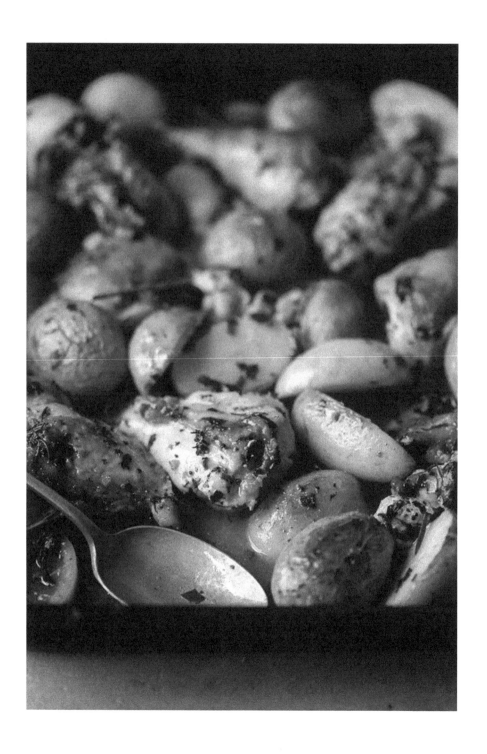

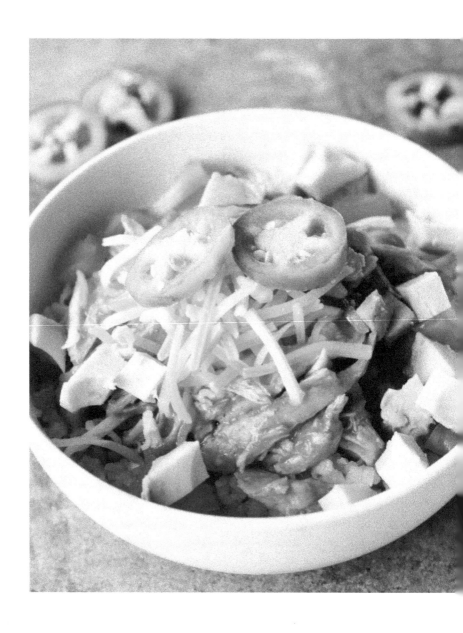

CPSIA information can be obtained
at www.ICGtesting.com
Printed in the USA
BVHW092304140621
609528BV00010B/1495